Beauty Smoothies

Green Smoothies for Youthful Skin, Vitality, Detox and Weight Management

Table of Contents

Buddy Banana Shake

Tangerine Dream

Classic Mango Lassi

Strawberry Orange Sunrise

Cocoa Avocado Smoothie

Watermelon Spritzer Smoothie

Bananarama Swirl

Apricot Peach Relief Mellow

Melon Morning Tropical Pop

Smoothie Lemon Squeeze

Tropical Spritzer Smoothie

Introduction

Everyone knows that the food people eat will directly affect their weight. It's pretty obvious, right? If you eat highly processed food, you gain weight. If you eat all natural healthy food, you lose weight and live a healthy life. It also gives your body the needed vitality to keep you strong in the face of life's stressful conditions.

The next question is can the food you eat give you youthful skin and help you detoxify? Now, that's an interesting proposition. Well, here's another question that may have tickled your fancy – can the food we eat affect our mood?

Improving Your Mood

Now that is also a very interesting thought. That is also one of the things that this book will teach you. Mood swings affect the way we approach life. It also affects our appetite. Scientists and diet experts have begun to see a connection between what a person eats and how that food affects a person's mood.

They also say that the food that we eat can change the chemicals that make our brain function. The food we eat can make us feel good about ourselves and it can give us a positive mental attitude. The information you'll find on this book will teach you how to choose and prepare food that will uplift your spirits.

Better Vitality and More Energy

To receive greater vitality, you need to stick to healthy natural food. Stay away from highly processed foods. To increase your body's vitality, you need to eat food that will serve as a natural source of energy. You're not going to get that from food that has a lot of processed sugar.

Loading up on glutinous food that has lots of sugar, which includes ice cream, cakes, and other pastries for instance, may seem like a quick fix when you need an energy boost, but that is not the way to go. You may have heard about cutting back on carbs but that doesn't mean you have to quit all forms of carbs.

There are carbs that are good for you and there are carbs that are harmful for the human body. What you really need to do is to cut back on processed carbs and stick to natural sources, which include fruits, legumes, and vegetables. These are all natural energy sources.

Getting Healthier Skin

Blemishes on the skin can be quite an annoyance. It's not only an issue for teenagers it's also a big concern for adults as well. Statistics also show that 20% of women who are already in their 30's and older still have skin blemishes.

Acne is not the only issue when it comes to getting healthier skin. Skin discolorations and other skin problems also become a huge concern. It's interesting that a natural approach to solve these skin problems is to simply make a few changes in one's diet.

Everyone wants a brighter and more radiant skin. Who wouldn't? It makes people feel good and it adds to their self-confidence. Now, the question is what sort of food do you need to get that radiant healthy skin?

Natural Food for Healthy Skin

It shouldn't be surprising that you don't really have to go far to find the food that will help improve your skin condition and give you generally better health. You don't need to buy any exotic food or go to some far away country to get that rare fruit that only grows in some unknown island somewhere in the world.

The only place you need to go to is the nearest grocery store where you can find the fruits and vegetables you need like tomatoes, kale, berries, radishes, red grapes, avocados, broccoli, hemp seeds, and brown rice. Take note that you want the natural ones, not the processed variants usually packed for your convenience.

Tomatoes are rich in nutrients that help protect your skin from the harmful rays of the sun. It's not a substitute for sunscreen but it helps make your skin stronger and more resistant.

Do you feel like you're having some sort of vitamin deficiency? Have some kale. Kale is considered by many dieters as a kind of super veggie. It has pretty much every nutrient needed by your body to stay healthy and fit. Kale not only makes you look beautiful, it also keeps you healthy.

If you want to get rid of skin blemishes as soon as possible, then add berries to your meal. Berries of different colors are recommended in this work. They're also a great solution for the many causes of acne.

Simply put, you need to make sure that your diet is free of processed foods. It should be gluten free, dairy free, and free of processed sugars.

Processed Foods Will Eventually Strain Your Body

Want to get rid of depression, improve skin condition, and live an energetic lifestyle? Then reduce (if you're not able to completely get rid of) processed foods in your life. Some have contemplated that processed foods are killing them one small bite (or extra bite if you sneak out to the fridge at night) at a time.

Let's face it. Processed foods are definitely a lot cheaper than whole foods that are much healthier. Organic foods are just a dollar or a few more dollars more expensive. But that's just a small cost compared to the destructive powers of processed food. Organic and natural foods are actually an investment not only in terms of dollars and cents but an investment in yourself – remember you are your best investment in life.

Take note that modified foods contain something called phosphates. Many processed foods have this type of chemical ingredient in them. They change the texture of the food, make it taste so much better, and extend the shelf life of these processed foods; but at what cost? They can cause rapid aging and some types of cancer.

Now you know why you have too many wrinkles at such a young age. Not only that; these phosphates also contribute to overall weakness in the bones and eventually kidney failure. So, give yourself a break – get rid of processed foods.

Processed Foods Are Addictive

Have you ever wondered why fast food is so hard to let go of? You can eat whole foods but you don't crave for them, right? You know they are good for you but you don't crave for them or wake up in the middle of the night just to have a bite of them.

The manufacturers of processed foods have included artificial ingredients that make the body crave for their products. These types of foods and food additives send signals of pleasure to the brain. Since your body only remembers very satisfying feelings after eating fast food and other forms of processed food, cravings will then overwhelm a person.

In the end, your brain is unable to resist the taste of processed sugar and processed salt. Do you wonder why that cheeseburger is addictive? What about the fries? What about that biggie sized soda? Yes, they have been chemically designed to become addictive. The secret is in the highly processed foods with laboratory produced ingredients that make you crave for these foods.

Can You Say Inflammation?

Inflammation is a plague in today's fast food society. Ever wonder why more and more people are getting the bulge? There's a reason why some people call processed foods as junk foods. They basically make your body bulge and that basically leads to problems in blood circulation, dementia, some breathing problems, and in worse case scenarios, some form of cancer.

Good Tasting Food from the Lab and Not the Farm

Most people think that their fries come from a farm somewhere. Wow, those fries are really huge! Oh yes, did you notice how tasty those burgers were? How about the chips in the bag?

They're so much better than the ones you have to peel and fry yourself, right? Have you ever wondered why that is so? It's because processed foods are most likely made out of GMOs. What's GMO? It's short for genetically modified organism; in short it's food grown in a lab and not some farm out there in the big wide open.

Going back to reality; every time you open your bag of chips, you should learn to visualize just where those chips came from. Even the breakfast cereals you eat have been exposed to more than 70 kinds of chemicals which include some pesticides as well.

Processed Foods Make You Obese

You may be wondering how processed food can make you obese. It's all because of that modified sugar known as fructose. If you care to check the label of processed food, you won't miss the fact that many of them contain some kind of fructose.

Sometimes it is fructose corn syrup and sometimes it's something else. But the bottom line is that it's all fructose. It's not real sugar but it's just an alternative to natural sugar.

Compared to sugar, fructose requires three times the processing time. This basically puts a lot of strain on your body. It takes the longest time for your body to digest it. Long story short, it just ends up getting stored as fat rather than being used next time you walk or take a hike to the office.

Raises Your Blood Sugar

Since we've already covered fructose, here are some more after effects that it will bring. Not only will it make people go obese, it also has an impact on your blood sugar. Taking in processed fructose is like throwing a wrench into a running engine; it will mess up your metabolism and eventually make your blood sugar go up real fast.

Real organic food and real natural sugar is the key to avoid all these problems. Remember that processed foods have a huge impact on your body. Your body will work at strained levels and result in a ruined mood and a bad outlook. You basically end up feeling bad inside and out.

Go Natural, Try Natural Smoothies

A steady growing body of scientific research is pointing to an obvious truth. And that is natural fruits and veggies tend to make you look and feel better. The research also shows that these foods are critical to promoting overall good health.

Natural foods contain all the essentials that your body needs to look good and make you feel better about yourself. They also act as a shield against many chronic diseases that many people suffer from today.

The idea is not to eat natural foods sparingly. You can't have processed foods as the main bulk of your diet and have a serving or two of fruits and veggies. Health experts have learned that people should eat generous servings of natural fruits and vegetables.

Another reason why you should be eating natural healthy foods is that they contain anti-oxidants. They basically detoxify your body and remove all the bad stuff that had been accumulated there over time. These anti-oxidants also have anti-aging properties that will make you look younger.

So why add smoothies to your diet? Unlike juices extracted from fruits and veggies, you don't throw the pulp away when you make a smoothie. The pulp is where a lot of the nutrients come from. That's basically where the health giving fiber is stored.

Smoothies are also easily digested. The food is already broken down into smaller particles, thus they are easier to ingest. That also makes them easier to digest – your tummy won't feel a thing.

Studies also show that smoothies are far better than juice extracts when it comes to weight loss. This is also due to the fiber content. Other than that, you also get a lot of raw vitamins and minerals from them.

You get mental clarity, you reduce the old cravings for processed food, and you immediately get a quick dose of energy boost. That's the power enough to boost your mood in spite of a busy life. Plus, smoothies are quick and easy to prepare. Have a natural fruit and veggie smoothie today.

Simple Almond Milk

Prep Time: 5 minutes*

Servings: 2

INGREDIENTS

1 cup raw almonds

4 cups water

INSTRUCTIONS

1. *Soak almonds in 1 cup water at least 6 hours, or overnight.
2. Drain soaked almonds and add to high-speed blender with 3 cups water. Process until well blended and almost smooth, about 1- 2 minutes.
3. Strain mixture through nutmilk bag, cheesecloth or strainer into container.
4. Keep refrigerated up to 4 days. If milk separates, mix before use.

Simple Coconut Milk

Prep Time: 10 minutes

Servings: 2

INGREDIENTS

2 mature coconuts

3 cups water

INSTRUCTIONS

1. Remove flesh from coconuts and add to high-speed blender with 3 cups water. Process until well blended and fairly smooth, about 1-2 minutes.
2. Strain mixture through nutmilk bag, cheesecloth or strainer into container.
3. Reserve pulp and set aside to dry and dehydrate, then use as coconut flour.
4. Keep refrigerated up to 4 days. If milk separates, mix before use.

NOTE: Blend additional coconut flesh with prepared coconut milk and strain forthicker coconut milk. Continue blending thickened coconut milk with additional coconut flesh until coconut cream forms.Or set thickened milk aside in refrigerator and allow fat to separate for coconut cream.

Dried Coconut Milk

Prep Time: 5 minutes*

Servings: 2

INGREDIENTS

2 cups dried coconut (unsweetened shreds or flakes)

4 cups of water

INSTRUCTIONS

1. *Soak dried coconut in 3 cups water at least 6 hours, or overnight in refrigerator.

2. Add soaked coconut and liquid to high-speed blender. Process until well blended and fairly smooth, about 1- 2 minutes. Add extra water for thinner consistency.

3. Strain mixture through nutmilk bag, cheesecloth or strainer into container.

4. Reserve pulp and set aside to dry and dehydrate, then use as coconut flour.

5. Keep refrigerated up to 4 days. If milk separates, mix before use.

NOTE: Increase coconut and decrease water for thicker coconut milk. Set thickened milk aside in refrigerator and allow fat to separate for coconut cream.

Super Green Smoothie

Prep Time: 5 minutes*

Servings: 1

INGREDIENTS

1 cup chopped kale

1/2 cup watercress

1 banana (frozen chunks)

1 green apple

1/2 avocado

1 1/2 cupsnut milk (or kefir)

2 - 4 tablespoons sweetener** (optional)

INSTRUCTIONS

1. *Peel banana, then chop and freeze.
2. Remove any stems and ribs from kale. Peel apple if preferred, then core and dice.
3. Slice avocado in half and scoop flesh of pitted half into high-speed blender. Add remaining ingredientsand process until smooth, about 1 - 2 minutes.
4. Pour into large glass and serve immediately.

**Stevia, dried dates or raw honey*

Emerald City Smoothie

Prep Time: 5 minutes

Servings: 1

INGREDIENTS

1 cup spinach

1 small zucchini (or 1/2 large)

2 celery stalks

1 cup green grapes

1 1/4 cupsnut milk

2 - 4 tablespoons sweetener* (optional)

INSTRUCTIONS

1. Peel zucchini if preferred, then chop. Chop celery stalks.
2. Add all ingredientsto high-speed blender. Process until smooth, about 1 - 2 minutes.
3. Pour into large glass and serve immediately.

*Stevia, dried dates or raw honey

Spiced PearPerfection

Prep Time: 5 minutes*

Servings: 1

INGREDIENTS

2 ripe pears

1 banana (frozen chunks)

1 1/4 cupsnut milk

1/2 teaspoon ground cinnamon

1/4teaspoon ground nutmeg

1/4 teaspoon vanilla

INSTRUCTIONS

1. *Peel banana, then cut into chucks and freeze.
2. Stem and seed pears, then cut into quarters.
3. Add all ingredients to high-speed blender. Process until smooth, about 1 minute.
4. Pour into large glass and serve immediately.

Ruby Slipper Smoothie

Prep Time: 5 minutes

Servings: 1

INGREDIENTS

1 cup strawberries (frozen halves)

1/2 cup red raspberries

1/2 cup pitted cherries

1 cupnut milk

1 tablespoon chia or flax seed (optional)

INSTRUCTIONS

1. *Remove stems from strawberries, then cut in half and freeze.
2. Pit cherries, if fresh.
3. Add frozen strawberries and nut milk to high-speed blender. Pulse to break down frozen strawberries.
4. Add remaining ingredients and process until smooth, about 1 minute.
5. Pour into large glass and serve immediately.

Strawberry Banana Mambo

Prep Time: 5 minutes*

Servings: 1

INGREDIENTS

1 banana (frozen chunks)

1 cup strawberries (frozen halves)

1 1/2 cupnut milk

1/4 teaspoon vanilla

INSTRUCTIONS

1. *Peel banana, then cut into chucks and freeze. Remove stems from strawberries, cut in half and freeze.
2. Add all ingredients to high-speed blender. Process until smooth, about 1- 2 minutes.
3. Pour into large glass and serve immediately.

Piña Colada Crush

Prep Time: 5 minutes*

Servings: 1

INSTRUCTIONS

1 small banana (frozen chunks)

1 cup pineapple (frozen chunks)

1 1/2 cupscoconut milk

2 tablespoons flaked coconut (or 1/4 cup fresh coconut)

DIRECTIONS

1. *Peel banana, then cut into chucks and freeze. Peel pineapple,then cut into chunks and freeze.
2. Add all ingredients to high-speed blender. Process until smooth, about 1- 2 minutes.
3. Pour into large glass and serve immediately.

Kiwi Strawberry Shake

Prep Time: 5 minutes*

Servings: 1

INGREDIENTS

1 cup strawberries (frozen halves)

2 kiwis

1cupnut milk

1/2 cup orange juice (about 2 oranges)

1 tablespoon chia or flax seed (optional)

INSTRUCTIONS

1. *Remove stems from strawberries, cut in half and freeze.
2. Peel kiwi and cut into quarters. Juice oranges.
3. Add all ingredients to high-speed blender. Process until smooth, about 1-2 minutes.
4. Pour into large glass and serve immediately.

Funny BunnySlushy

Prep Time: 10 minutes*

Servings: 1

INGREDIENTS

1 small banana (frozen chunks)

1/2 cup pineapple (frozen chunks)

2 large carrots

Small pieceginger root

1/2 cuporange juice (about 2 oranges)

1 cupnut milk

1/2 teaspoon ground cinnamon

1 cage-free egg (optional)

INSTRUCTIONS

1. *Peel banana, then cut into chucks and freeze. Peel pineapple,then cut into chunks and freeze.

2. Juice carrots, oranges and ginger root.

3. Add all ingredients to high-speed blender. Process until smooth, about 1- 2 minutes.

4. Pour into large glass and serve immediately.

Chunky Monkey Smoothie

Prep Time: 5 minutes

Servings: 1

INGREDIENTS

1 large banana (or 2 small)

2 tablespoonsraw cocoa powder

1 cupnut milk

1/2 cup ice

2 - 4 tablespoons sweetener* (optional)

INSTRUCTIONS

1. Peel and chop banana.
2. Add ice and nut milk to high-speed blender. Pulse to crush ice.
3. Add remainingingredients and process until smooth, about 1- 2 minutes.
4. Pour into large glass and serve immediately.

*Stevia, dried dates or raw honey

Cucumber MelonSwirl

Prep Time: 5 minutes*

Servings: 2

INGREDIENTS

1 small cucumber

1 cup watermelon (chunks)

1 cup honeydew melon (frozen chunks)

1 cupcoconut milk

2 - 4 tablespoons sweetener** (optional)

INSTRUCTIONS

1. * Cut honeydew flesh away from peel, then cut into chunks and freeze.
2. Peel cucumber and remove seeds, then cut into chunks. Cut watermelon flesh away from rind, then remove seeds and cut into chunks.
3. Add all ingredients to high-speed blender. Process until smooth, about 1 minute.
4. Pour into large glasses and serve immediately.

Stevia, dried dates or raw honey

All-Star Strawberry Smoothie

Prep Time: 5 minutes*

Servings: 1

INGREDIENTS

1 cup strawberries

1 cup strawberries (frozen halves)

2 cupscoconut milk

1/2 teaspoon vanilla

2 tablespoons chia or flax seed (optional)

INSTRUCTIONS

1. * Remove stems from 1 cup strawberries, then cut in half and freeze.
2. Remove stems from 1 cup fresh strawberries.
3. Add frozen strawberries and coconut milk to high-speed blender. Pulse to break down frozen strawberries.
4. Add remainingingredients and process until smooth, about 1- 2 minutes.
5. Pour into large glass and serve immediately.

Banana Berry Bliss

Prep Time: 5 minutes*

Servings: 1

INGREDIENTS

1 banana (frozen chunks)

1/2 cup strawberries (frozen halves)

1/4 cup blueberries

1/4 cup blackberries

1 1/2 cups nut milk

1/2 teaspoon vanilla

2 tablespoons chia or flax seed (optional)

INSTRUCTIONS

1. *Peel banana, then cut into chucks and freeze. Remove stems from strawberries,then cut in half and freeze.
2. Add all ingredients to high-speed blender. Process until smooth, about 1 - 2 minutes.
3. Pour into large glass and serve immediately.

Blue Sapphire Smoothie

Prep Time: 5 minutes

Servings: 1

INGREDIENTS

1 cup blueberries (frozen)

1/4 cup black raspberries

1/4 cup blackberries

1/4 cup pitted black cherries

1 /2 cups nut milk

1/2 teaspoon vanilla

2 tablespoons chia or flax seed (optional)

INSTRUCTIONS

1. *Freeze blueberries.
2. Add alls ingredients to high-speed blender. Process until smooth, about 1minute.
3. Pour into large glass and serve immediately.

Nutty Buddy Banana Shake

Prep Time: 5 minutes*

Servings: 1

INGREDIENTS

1 banana (frozen chunks)

1/4 cup raw almond butter (or 1/2 cup raw almonds)

1cupnut milk

2 - 4 tablespoons sweetener**

INSTRUCTIONS

1. *Peel banana, then cut into chucks and freeze.
2. Add raw almonds to food processor or high speed blender and process until smooth, about 3 minutes. Or use prepared raw almond butter.
3. Add all ingredients to high-speed blender. Process until smooth, about 1 - 2 minutes.
4. Pour into large glass and serve immediately.

*Stevia, dried dates or raw honey

Tangerine Dream

Prep Time: 5 minutes

Servings: 1

INGREDIENTS

1 1/2 cupsorange or tangerine juice (about 6 oranges or 10 tangerines)

1/2cup coconutcream (or thick coconut milk)

2/3 cup ice

1 cage-free egg (optional)

2 tablespoons sweetener* (optional)

INSTRUCTIONS

1. Juice oranges.

2. Add ice and orange juice to high-speed blender. Pulse to crush ice.

3. Add remaining ingredients and process until smooth, about 1minute.

4. Pour into large glass and serve immediately.

*Stevia, dried dates or raw honey

Classic Mango Lassi

Prep Time: 5 minutes

Servings: 1

INGREDIENTS

1 ripe mango

1 cupcoconut milk

1/2 cup ice

1 cage-free egg (optional)

2 - 4 tablespoons sweetener* (optional)

INSTRUCTIONS

1. Cut flesh of mango from pit. Remove peel and cut into chunks.
2. Add ice and coconut milk to high-speed blender. Pulse to crush ice.
3. Add remaining ingredients and process until smooth, about 1 minute.
4. Pour into large glass and serve immediately.

*Stevia, dried dates or raw honey

Strawberry Orange Sunrise

Prep Time: 5 minutes*

Servings: 1

INGREDIENTS

1 cupstrawberries

1/2 cup strawberries (frozen halves)

1 cup orange juice (about 4 oranges)

1/2 cup thick coconut milk(or kefir)

2 tablespoons chia or flax seed (optional)

INSTRUCTIONS

1. *Remove stems from 1/2 cup strawberries,then cut in half and freeze.
2. Remove stem from fresh strawberries. Juice oranges
3. Add frozen strawberries and orange juice to high-speed blender. Pulse to break downfrozen strawberries.
4. Add remaining ingredients and process until smooth, about 1 minute.
5. Pour into large glass and serve immediately.

Cocoa Avocado Smoothie

Prep Time: 5 minutes

Servings: 1

INGREDIENTS

1 ripe avocado

1 cupcoconut milk (or kefir)

1/3 cup ice

1/2 teaspoon vanilla

2 - 4 tablespoons sweetener*

2 tablespoons raw cocoa powder (optional)

INSTRUCTIONS

1. Add ice and coconut milk to high-speed blender. Pulse to crush ice.

2. Slice avocado in half and remove pit. Scoop into high-speed blender.

3. Add remaining ingredients and process until smooth, about 1 minute.

4. Pour into large glass and serve immediately.

*Stevia, dried dates or raw honey

Watermelon Spritzer Smoothie

Prep Time: 5 minutes*

Servings: 1

INGREDIENTS

2 cups watermelon (chunks)

1/2 cup strawberries (frozen halves)

2 limes

1/2 cupthick coconut milk

2 - 4 tablespoons sweetener**

INSTRUCTIONS

1. *Remove stems from strawberries, then cut in halve and freeze.
2. Cut watermelon flesh away from rind and cut into chunks. Juice limes.
3. Add frozen strawberries, lime juice and nut milk to high-speed blender. Pulse to break down frozen strawberries.
4. Add all ingredients and to high-speed blender. process until smooth, about 1 minute.
5. Pour into large glass and serve immediately.

**Stevia, dried dates or raw honey

BananaramaSwirl

Prep Time: 5 minutes*

Servings: 1

INGREDIENTS

1 banana (frozen chunks)

1 plum

1/4 cup pitted prunes

1 cupnut milk

1/2 cup orange juice (about 2 oranges)

1 cage-free egg (optional)

INSTRUCTIONS

1. *Peel banana, then cut into chucks and freeze.
2. Cut plum in half and remove pit, then quarter. Juice oranges.
3. Add all ingredients to high-speed blender. Process until smooth, about 1 - 2 minutes.
4. Pour into large glass and serve immediately.

Apricot Peach Relief

Prep Time: 5 minutes

Servings: 1

INGREDIENTS

1 ripe peach or nectarine (frozen chunks)

2 fresh apricots (or 1/4 cup dried)

1/2 cup nut milk (or kefir)

1/2 cup fresh orange juice (about 2 oranges)

1 cage-free egg (optional)

INSTRUCTIONS

1. *Cut peach in half and remove pit, then cut into chucks and freeze.
2. Cut fresh apricots in half and remove pits, then cut into chucks, if using. Juice oranges.
3. Add all ingredients to high-speed blender. Process until smooth, about 1 minute.
4. Pour into large glass and serve immediately.

Mellow Melon Morning

Prep Time: 5 minutes*

Servings: 1

INGREDIENTS

1 cup honeydew melon (frozen chunks)

1 cup cantaloupe (chunks)

1 grapefruit (about 2/3 cup juice)

2/3 cupthick coconut milk

2 - 4 tablespoons sweetener**

INSTRUCTIONS

1. *Cut honeydew melon flesh away from rind,then cut into chunks and freeze.

2. Cut cantaloupe flesh away from rind,then cut into chunks.Juice grapefruit.

3. Add frozen honeydew chunks and grapefruit juice to high-speed blender. Pulse to break down frozen honeydew.

4. Add remaining ingredients and process until smooth, about 1 minute.

5. Pour into large glass and serve immediately.

**Stevia, dried dates or raw honey

Tropical Pop Smoothie

Prep Time: 5 minutes

Servings: 1

INGREDIENTS

1 mango (frozen chunks)

1/2 cup papaya (chunks)

1 ripe guava

2 limes

1 cupcoconut milk

INSTRUCTIONS

1. *Cut mango flesh away from pit and peel. Then dice into small chunks and freeze.
2. Peel papaya and remove seeds, then cut into chunks. Peel guava if preferred, then cut in half. Juice limes.
3. Add coconut milk and guava to high-speed blender. Process until smooth. Strain out seeds, reserving liquid.
4. Add strained guava mixture back to high-speed blender with frozen mango chunks. Pulse to break down frozen mango.
5. Add remaining ingredients and process until smooth, about 1 minute.
6. Pour into large glass and serve immediately.

Lemon Squeeze

Prep Time: 5 minutes

Servings: 1

INGREDIENTS

1/2 cup fresh lemon juice (about 3 lemons)

1/2 cup fresh orange juice (about 2 oranges)

1/2 cup coconut milk

1/2 cupice

2 - 4 tablespoons sweetener*

INSTRUCTIONS

1. Juice lemons and oranges.
2. Add ice and coconut milk to high-speed blender. Pulse to crush ice.
3. Add remaining ingredients and process until smooth, about 1 minute.
4. Pour into large glass and serve immediately.

*Stevia, dried dates or raw honey

Tropical Spritzer Smoothie

Prep Time: 5 minutes

Servings: 1

INGREDIENTS

1/2 cup lime juice (about 5 limes) 1 sprig fresh mint

1/2 cup thick coconut milk

2 tablespoons flaked coconut (or 1/4 cup fresh coconut)

1/2 cup ice

2 - 4 tablespoons sweetener*

1/2 teaspoon vanilla

(optional)

INSTRUCTIONS

1. Remove mint leaves from stem. Juice limes.
2. Add ice and limes juice to high-speed blender. Pulse to crush ice.
3. Add remaining ingredients to high-speed blender and process until smooth, about 1 minute.
4. Pour into large glass and serve immediately.

*Stevia, dried dates or raw honey

www.ingramcontent.com/pod-product-compliance
Lightning Source LLC
Chambersburg PA
CBHW070132290526
45789CB00005B/2210